I0840156

THE COMMON SENSE KETO DIET.

BEGINNER'S GUIDE, WITH SIMPLE AND EFFECTIVE STEPS TO KETO MADE DIET FOR WEIGHT LOSS

By

James Young

Table of Contents

Copyright©2019

And it is punishable by law. Do not participate in or
Encourage electronic piracy of copyrighted material.

DISCLAIMER

This publication is designed to provide competent and
reliable information regarding the subject matter. However, it is sold with the understanding that the author is not engaged in rendering professional advice. If an expert assistance is required, the services of a professional should Be Sought.
The author specifically negate any liability that is incurred from the use or application of the Contents of this material.

Introduction

The ketogenic diet was introduced between 1920s-

30s to help curb seizures in epileptic children.

This diet will force the body to burn fat instead of carbohydrates, because the carbohydrates in the food is converted into glucose which is specifically substantial for charging the brain. However, the Liver converts fat into fatty acid and ketone bodies which replaces glucose as an energy source.

These ketone bodies leads to drastic decline in Prevalence of epileptic seizures.

In the 1970s, the ketogenic diet started gaining abundant concentration as a promising weight-loss strategy due to Low-Carb diet trend. Today, the ketogenic diet is distinguished for its extraordinary

High-fat content with moderate protein intake.

In this cookbook:

• You'll be exposed to varieties of ketogenic

   Recipes.

• You'll learn how to prepare these recipes with step

   By step guide.

• You'll also be exposed to pocket friendly and

   Readily available recipes.

And much more!

Without further ado, let's dive right into it.

What is a Ketogenic diet?

A Ketogenic Diet is any diet that helps you produce more ketones. Usually, the liver is responsible for this.

The body usually likes to feed on glucose and use it as fuel. When you consume a high carb diet it prefers the
former, when this isn't available, the body tend to shift its fuel grabbing attention to fats. This activity is what induces ketosis.

Ketosis is the process of making fuel with fats available rather than the carbs which are pretty limited or absent. This serves as a way to control your blood sugar.

Initially when you feed on carbs, insulin is produced and sugar is released and used by the body. Due to high level of insulin, fats are stored.

When you enter the state of ketosis, there is a limited amount of carbs and a low insulin level.

Due to this low insulin level, more fats are demanded from storage areas and used up.

A process known as ketosis and carried out by the action of the liver.

As these sugar levels are controlled, there is less cravings. Again when you add a protein to the diet, you will feel satisfied. So hereby leading to less hunger.

Types of keto diet

The keto diet is a wonder diet, especially if you have been searching for a convenient way to reach ketosis faster. We shall discuss briefly some of the types of keto diet and how they affect your overall lifestyle.

Standard ketogenic diet

This diet contains keto macros in the following ratio: 75% fat,15-20% protein, 5-10% carbs

Most diet containing the standard diet of keto is arranged around the following meals and specific examples are avocados, butter, ghee, fatty fish and meats, olives and olive oil. Remember that eating about 150 grams will enable your body system begins to shift its focus from carbs dependency to burning fat for fuel. So when you are working on the keto diet, there is a need to cut down on carbs. If you have been used to eating around 300 grams of carbs per day , now is the time you should slash it down to about 50 grams of carbs per Day. Next we have another type of keto diet .

Targeted keto diet (TKD)

In this diet , there is an easy sharing formula for our macros. It depends on the following ratio: 65-70% fat, 20% protein, 10-15% carbs

Athletes will find this diet useful.

They are usually able to keep a constant check on their lifestyle. A daily carb intake of about 30 grams might be optimal for their lifestyle the will mostly consume grain based foods and sports products. Most additional carbs will be burned off as fuel since they are an active group of people.

Cyclical keto diet (CKD)

This diet has a keto macros ratio of: 75% fat, 15-20% protein, 5-10% carbs on keto days; 25% fat, 25% protein and 50% carbs on off days.

This is a time where you are off the keto diet balance. You enter and after some weeks you take some days off.

Some prefer to do this during the holiday. So the cycling is actually a time of being off and on.

High-Protein Keto Diet

The Macronutrient ratio of the high protein keto diet is: 60-65% fat, 30% protein, 5-10% carb.

In this plan you require about 120grams of protein every day and 130 grams of fat per day. The carbs are now limited to around 10% of the total ratio.

Many people love this keto diet because they prefer to eat a high protein content meal than a standard fat containing meal of Ketogenic diet.

The effect of this preference is delay in reaching ketosis faster.

There is no preferred type of keto diet that's the best. You need to begin and keep records of your progress. That is what this book is all about.

What kind of food should we eat?

Since the Ketogenic diet limits carbohydrate intake to a certain amount per day, it's expected that you will start with the suggested amount of 20g every day. This will remove any unwanted carbs and other fat inducing carbs. In order to determine the net carbs, we shall move the overall carbs from fibre carbs. You can and should be getting your carbs from any of the following as vegetables, nuts, dairy, avoid carbs that have been refined like bread.

You should set a daily carbs target you plan to reach. Anything you eat should fall within either a protein or fat.
We hope you will get into ketosis early enough to reach that precious goal.
So whenever you go shopping and Purchase some food item, read the labels carefully. You want to be sure there is nothing that is off limits which may affect your diet plan.

When you eat enough protein, it will affect your muscle build up. This should be encouraged. The reason why is that we are trying to shed fat but we shouldn't limit it to that, Build those muscles for it will be a wonderful thing for you to do.
Importance of keto macros
The Ketogenic diet really can take some time and the process is not really smooth at the initial stages. A lot of things happen. Your liver is under a

constant work of producing ketones and you need to keep some level of balance. This balance is achieved when you know the correct macros for this process. Many studies and experts has revealed that the ratio of carbs to protein to fat should be 60%-35%-5%. This is not an accurate way or method but it's still helpful.
You should aim to reach a carb goal of 20g each day.

Should I count calories or not?

People love to track their progress and results. So therefore counting the amount of calories may be useful if you need to know when and how progress is made when you are on the Ketogenic diet. You may track your progress manually. it's advisable and the right thing to do.

How will I feel as I make progress?

You will feel lots of disruption from your normal self. Things such as nausea, headaches, dizziness, mental fog with flu-like symptoms also known as keto flu.

They will all happen. You can't take anything away from it.

Don't worry, Relax. That's how we all felt in this so you aren't alone.

 The Ketogenic diet is basically carried out by the liver. The liver produces the ketones and aids the process greatly. You may find that you don't have as much endurance and strength as used to, and this is normal. So your body begins to use fat as fuel. With time , you shall become stable .

How to test for ketones

There are three common ways you can test for ketones, namely...

• Breath Test(using Ketonix meter)

• Using blood ketone meter

• Urine Test(using ketone urine strips). For the purpose of this lesson, we shall concentrate on Urine test. This is because, the Ketone Urine strips are very easy to use and also pocket friendly.

The Urine test is carried out by dipping the Ketone Urine strips into urine, you'll notice some shadows of a pink or purple colours depending on the degree of ketone at that moment.

Further research shows that, ketone urine test is likely to be top-notch when carried out early in the morning and after dinner while on ketogenic diet.

So, when next you need to have a checkup on your progress, you can give the urinary ketone test a try.

Benefits of keto diet

There are some aspects of the keto diet that are always being debated.

There have been major concerns about consuming a high fat meal.

Will this not lead to an increase in cholesterol or other heart related disease?

However, in most scientific studies, low-carb diets prove their worth as healthy and beneficial.

A low carb diet also prevents and affects the build up of harmful fats as only the needed fatty acids are used and produced. This will also affect heart diseases — including cholesterol.

Now let's consider some of the health benefits of cholesterol.The keto diet helps control your hunger, It's no longer news that hunger is not a very good thing as it causes more adverse effect to us. So when you are on a high fat low carb diet, you hunger tends to be controlled and this is a good sign.

Scientific studies revealed that people who take a low carb diet needs fewer calories each day.

So reducing your carb intake will also affect your appetite as it will be cut down. Again low carb diet will help you lose weight.

Removes excess water from the body

As you feed on the low carb diets as specified in this guide, you will tend to lose weight faster. There is also an increase in water loss. They lose water too.

Since where fats are stored in your body determines the type of diseases that arises from the body. Most people who are on the keto diet lose abdominal fat. In essence, low carb diets helps immediate weight loss.

So getting rid of this abdominal or visceral fat is vital to a healthy lifestyle. This is the target of most men on this diet.

Removal of harmful triglycerides

Triglycerides are the harmful fatty acids we do not want. They tend to trigger some heart disease especially when one is on a high carbs. Having a low carb diet eliminates this.

Increased Levels High-density lipoprotein (HDL) or "good" cholesterol.

 A high fat low carb diet will increase the levels of these lipoprotein and promote healthy cholesterol levels.

Lower Blood Sugar and Insulin Levels

Lower the blood sugar levels. This is particularly useful for those with diabetes and related disease.

 If you are on blood sugar medication, you need to consult your doctor before you make any adjustments to your carb intake. This will help to prevent any disease

Reduction in the intake of carbs will lead to a reduction in sugar level and insulin level and this is a positive factor for those having type2 diabetes.

Lowers Blood Pressure

When someone has a hypertensive health or high blood pressure, this is a sign that there are underlying diseases present in the body system.

Therefore its normal after some time on a high fat low carb diet, many of the symptoms will reduce. The blood pressure begins to go down along with other associated health risk.

How do I Control Carbs Cravings?

Yes, cravings are real. They do occur. Our body system is a dynamic system and it can adapt to changes.

Due to the love for carbs and sugar, when you begin to cut down on these, your body may begin to crave carbs. This can be controlled.

You need to be firm in your resolve to stick to the Ketogenic diet plan. When you decided to go on a low carb diet.

You chose to take the risk. The risk is what's causing these.
Never ever give in, hang on a while and your body will naturally adapt to the new diet program.

A very effective method I adopted in controlling carbs cravings was "DISTRACTION". What I usually do, is to grab my game pad or play mind games. It was immensely helpful.

keypoint

The Ketogenic diet is a healthy diet that has been medically proven to be commendable for those that engage in it for one reason or the other. Be it weight loss, healthy cooking or living healthy. Prepare the meals you will find in this book with confidence and get ready to shed some pounds in a matter of weeks. Now that we've established what ketosis is, let's get into the kitchen and prep some delicious recipes.

Chapter one.
Steak and eggs.

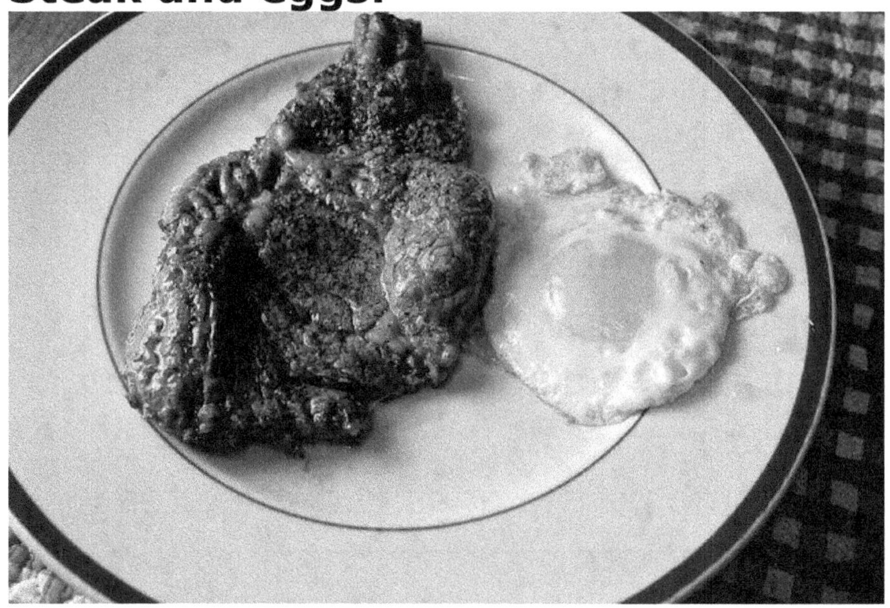

The finished recipes

How to prepare:

Put all vegetables aside and prepare them Cut the onions and pepper, preheat your bacon grease and be sure it's quite hot

Then begin to fry.

After this, it is time to do the steak .For this steak, after three minutes of cooking, you turn it aside and cook again for three minutes

There are no fast rules. Get an amount of steak you really need depending on the servings.

Now that the steak is done, it is time to make the eggs.

Now it's time for the scrambled eggs part. Get some eggs and use a scrambler, get them scrambled. After this is done, add some cheese and stir as desired.

Now combine the eggs with the steak

Information:

Serves: 10
Serving size: 362 g
Calories: 506
Fat: 51
Carbohydrates: 4
Fiber: 1

Protein: 45

Prep time: 10 mins
Cook time: 15 mins
Total time: 25 mins

Ingredients:
1 Onion (270 g)

1 Pepper (180 g)
4 lbs Beef Chuck Shoulder
15 Eggs
120 g Heavy Cream
5 Oz Cheddar Cheese
Salt, Pepper, Onion Powder, Garlic
Powder to taste

Chapter two

Tequila Chicken

Tequila Chicken Information:

Serves: 6
Serving size: 1 Breast
Calories: 445
Fat: 22
Carbohydrates: 2
Fiber: 0
Protein: 60

Prep time: 3 hours 15 mins
Cook time: 23 mins
Total time: 3 hours 38 mins
Ingredients:
Marinade

1 Cup Water
¼ Cup Soy Sauce
2 Tbsp. Lime Juice
½ tsp Garlic Powder
½ tsp Liquid Smoke
½ tsp Salt
50 mL Tequila (1 Shot)
6 Chicken Breasts
Sauce

¼ Cup Mayonnaise

¼ Cup Sour Cream

¼ Cup Tomato Sauce (or Salsa)

1 tsp. Heavy Cream

¼ tsp Dried Parsley

¼ tsp Frank's Hot Sauce

¼ tsp Salt

¼ tsp Dried Dill

¼ tsp Paprika

¼ tsp Cayenne Pepper

¼ tsp Ground Cumin

¼ tsp Chilli Powder

¼ tsp Black Pepper

6 oz. Cheddar Cheese, shredded

How To Prepare-:

Get a bowl and mix all marinade
ingredients together
Now add your chicken breast and
refrigerate for two to three hours
Remove from the refrigerator and get
anew broiler pan. Broil for about

twenty minutes. Flipping in between them

Test and see if the meat is ready. We are using 165 degrees heat

Get a dish and place your meat inside it. Add cheese to this

Broil at the same temperature until the meal is ready for serving.

Chapter three.

Baked Egg

The recipe Information.

Serves: 2
Serving size: ½
Calories: 337
Fat: 24
Carbohydrates: 5
Fiber: 1
Protein: 23

Prep time: 10 mins
Cook time: 25 mins
Total time: 35 mins

Ingredients:

4 Eggs

4 Slices Bacon
Salt and Pepper to taste
1 Oz Cheddar
1 Small Onion (80g)

Preparation How To Prepare-

Preheat the oven and be ready to fry the bacon

Get a bacon and put inside the pan then fry them for some time

Again you should Cut an onion and fry for some time

Now place the bacon with the onions inside a bowl

Get some eggs, two preferably and crack them without breaking the yoke.

Put in some salt and pepper

Add cheddar cheese

Heat at 350 degrees for 20 minutes until you see the eggs setting

Chapter four.

Reuben Casserole

Reuben Casserole Nutrition Information:

Serves: 4

Serving size: 1/4th
Calories: 769
Fat: 63
Carbohydrates: 10
Fiber: 4
Protein: 37

Prep time: 10 mins
Cook time: 35 mins
Total time: 45 mins
Ingredients:

12 Oz. Cooked Corned Beef
68 g Onion (1 Small)
1 can Sauerkraut (14.5 Oz)
8 Oz. Carlsberg
4 Oz. Cheddar Cheese
½ Cup Thousand Island Dressing
¼ Cup Mayo
Pepper to taste

How To Prepare-

Get a large bowl. You will need to slice corn beef inside this.
Get corn beef and slice them as desired into this bowl
Get some onions and a grater and chop the onions with this accordingly
Carlsberg is necessary at this point. We need to shred this with the grater too. Now use the large opening side to this and begin shredding the Carlsberg add a can of Sauerkraut   to the bowl.

Now it's the time to put the cheese to the bowl. Get some cheddar cheese and put them inside the bowl too.
Measure out ½ cup Thousand Island Dressing and ¼ cup Mayo and add to the bowl
Add fresh pepper to taste
Mix, then spread into a greased, 8" pan
Bake at 350 degrees for 35 minutes

Chapter five.

Juicy Lucy Sliders.

**Juicy Lucy Sliders!
Nutrition Information**

Serves: 4
Serving size: 1 burger
Calories: 285

Fat: 21
Carbohydrates: 0
Fiber: 0
Protein: 22

Prep time: 25 mins
Cook time: 5 mins
Total time: 30 mins

Ingredients:

1 lb. 6 oz. Ground Beef
1 Egg
Garlic / Salt / Pepper / Onion Powder to
taste
Several dashes of Worcestershire
Sauce
8 oz. Cheddar Cheese (1/2 oz. per
patty)

How To Prepare-
Get a bowl for this , there are a number
of things to mix up immediately.

Get the beef, eggs and spices and mix them together. The beef has to be sliced as desired and in the normal quantity you need

cut the meat and Divide them into 1.5 oz. patties

now Add ½ oz. of cheese to each Combine both of them to make a burger.

Now use both hands and press them together

Preheat the oven at 350 degrees, pour some oil in it and fry the burger. watch carefully and when done . remove from heat

You can always top up with cheese.

Chapter six.

Chocolate Strawberry Mousse

Nutrition Information

Serves: 1
Serving size: 105 g
Calories: 330
Fat: 33

Carbohydrates: 12

Fiber: 1
Protein: 10

Prep time: 3 mins
Cook time: 2 mins
Total time: 5 mins

Ingredients

⅓ Cup Heavy Whipping Cream

4 Drops EZ-Sweet
1 Strawberry (24g)
½ Scoop Chocolate Whey Powder (14g)

2.5 g Unsweetened Cocoa

Flakes of 90% Chocolate.

How To Prepare-

Get a container that wide enough and be ready to prepare this recipe. We are going to be mixing up a lot of things
Pour an ample amount of cream into the bowl and move to the next step.
Depending on the type you have purchased, add the liquid sweetener.
Now it's the time to Add the strawberry to our mix
Add your powder
Add the chocolate flakes you have got
Mix them up for 1-2 minutes or until the dough becomes thickened
Serve! For 2 0r three as desired

Chapter seven.

Blackened Pork Chops

Nutrition Information

Serves: 4
Serving size: 1 Chop (210g)
Calories: 341
Fat: 15

Carbohydrates: 4

Fiber: 1

Protein: 46

Prep time: 5 mins
Cook time: 10 mins
Total time: 15 mins

Ingredients:

4 Pork Chops (842 g)

1 Tbsp. Paprika

2 tsp Salt

1 tsp Garlic Powder

1 tsp Onion Powder

¼ tsp Cayenne Pepper

2 tsp Black Pepper

½ tsp Thyme Leaves

½ tsp Oregano Leaves

1 tsp Cumin

4 Tbsp. Butter

How To Prepare-:

Now you have a list of ingredients.
Gather the ingredients in a small sized
bowl.

Using a second bowl, melt four tablespoon of butter.

Preheat the oven and put some bacon grease then heat them up
Pick any of the chopped ingredients and dip in our melted butter, coat them up with some spice before dropping in the pan
Repeat the same process for some time until all have been done
Cook for 3-5 minutes on each side then flip to the other side
Cook until ready to serve
Note: Try reducing the amount of spices since it contains carbs and we are going on Ketogenic diet.

Chapter eight.

Cameroons Brochette.

Stuffed and Wrapped Shrimp
Nutrition Information

Serves: 4

Serving size: 4 Shrimp

Calories: 252

Fat: 15

Carbohydrates: 3

Fiber: 1

Protein: 28

Prep time: 5 mins
Cook time: 10 mins
Total time: 15 mins

Ingredients

1.5 lbs Large, cooked, peeled and deveined shrimp

15 slices Bacon

1 Tbsp. Garlic Powder

1 Tbsp. Pepper

1 Tbsp. Paprika

¼ tsp Cayenne Pepper

15 Jalapeno Slices

5 Slices Cheddar Cheese

How To Prepare-

Get a new bowl or a clean one and be ready to mix
Ensure that shrimp has been unfrozen and ready to be used
Mix all four major ingredients in the bowl
Dry shrimp and separate three quarters of it. We shall use this as desired
Open the shrimps. You need to put some cheese and jalapeno spice inside it
Cut the bacon into half and wrap the shrimp with them. Leave a space I the middle
Now gradually Skew shrimp as desired
Put them in the oven at 360 degrees and cook until it becomes crisps
desired

Chapter nine.

Keto Cocktails: Keto Margarita.

Prep time: 5 mins
Total time: 5 mins
Ingredients

1 Lime
1.5 oz. Tequila
4 drops Sucralose

How To Prepare-

You need some lime well cut and juiced. Then pour the juice in a container.

Get a glass cup and fill it with crushed or regular ice as you deem fit

add 1 jigger (1.5 oz.) of lime juice into glass

take some (1.5 oz.) of tequila and add them into glass cup

now we shall add 4 drops Sucralose

stir them all . now you can garnish
with a slice of lime

Chapter ten.

Eggs in a Cloud

Nutrition Information

Serves: 4
Serving size: 1
Calories: 98
Fat: 7
Carbohydrates: 1
Fiber: 0
Protein: 6

Prep time: 5 mins
Cook time: 5 mins
Total time: 10 mins

Ingredients

4 Large Eggs
2 Slices Bacon
To Taste Salt, Pepper, Onion Powder,
Garlic Powder
2 Tbsp. Parmesan Cheese

How To Prepare-

Break some eggs and separate the yolk
from the egg whites
Cut in pieces some bacon and cook
until it becomes brown
Get a good bowl, out the eggs in it.
Whip with a good blender until it
becomes stiff. Then set it aside
  Parmesan cheese should be added
into the egg white with bacon
  Using parchment paper, pour some
amount of egg white on it and form

mounds with them. Repeat the same process until you now have four mounds.
Bake the egg whites at 350 degrees for 5 minutes until they are set
Add the egg yolk into each mound
Bake for some time till you notice a brown colour

Chapter eleven.

Bacon Weave Sandwich.

 You need four bacon slices.
After getting them, you slice them into four pieces. And three sections in each piece. So we now have 12 slices
Cut them into three equal sections, you will now it's time to weave the slice.
Ensure that the kind of bacon you have is very strong for the bread so that it sticks together for the purpose we want to use it for.
Tools:

Cast iron griddle

Beacon press

Fish spatula

 The process:

Now move the bacon weave to the griddle and ensure that the bacon weave stays in one place as intended.

 While this is going on eggs can be cooked.

Preheat the bacon weave with the eggs. You will notice that it attaches itself.

Ensure that the egg is cracked into a bowl

Just for kicks, I used the egg form to cut out the cheese so it fit perfectly. Preheat at 360 for 5 minutes and allow to be done and ready for serving.

Chapter twelve

Bacon Brussels sprouts

Information:

Serves: 4

Serving size: 1/4th

Calories: 143

Fat: 10

Carbohydrates: 8

Fiber: 3

Protein: 6

Prep time: 10 mins
Cook time: 40 mins
Total time: 50 mins
List of Ingredients:

24 Oz Brussels Sprouts

¼ Cup Fish Sauce

¼ Cup Bacon Grease (Can substitute any oil)

6 Strips Bacon (Optional)

To Taste Pepper

How To Prepare-

Remove Brussels sprouts from stems and prepare them

Get a preparation bowl and get ready to mix a number of the ingredients

Prepare a fish sauce for the purpose of our recipe

Mix these: Brussels sprouts with the bacon grease and fish sauce all in the bowl

All the bacon to cook and begin to cut them into smaller strips

Add some bacon mix them together in the mix   and stir

Now bring out the Brussels sprouts and lay on a greased pan

Heat oven at 450 degrees for 40 minutes, and begin cooking while you stir every 10 minutes

Finally you should Finish off on broiling for a few minutes

Chapter thirteen.

Cast Iron Skillet Frittata

We need to begin cooking the bacon for this recipe. But first get the vegetables needed and prepare them.

Now get the green pepper and onions and begin slicing them . Make them look crisp because they need to appear fine when fried

Gather all the Brussels sprouts and soak them in a separate bowl. Allow it to soak for sometime.

Use a food processor and slice the Brussel sprouts. While you are getting them sliced, your bacon should be about ready for the next step.Now throw all the vegetables in and fry them too with your bacon

While they are getting fried, I threw in some week's cheddar. Actually, I am preparing this on the side.

 Now we shall pick 12 eggs, and mix them in 180 ml of heavy cream   with spices.

Whisk the eggs and put it aside.

Next, add the bacon to the mixture and do not allow the cheese in there for too long

Mix them all,

Cook for two to three minutes so you will set the bottom of the mixture. We do not want a running frittata
Preheat your oven and cook for 25 minutes. After some time, we now have our Cast Iron Skillet Frittata.

Nutritional Information:

Serves: 8
Serving size: 1/8the
Calories: 491
Fat: 35
Carbohydrates: 18
Fiber: 6
Protein: 29

Prep time: 20 mins
Cook time: 50 mins
Total time: 1 hour 10 mins

List of Ingredients:

8 Slices Bacon
1 Small Onion (125 g)
1 Small Pepper (133 g)
542 g Brussels Sprouts
1 Head Cauliflower (965 g)
12 Oz. Cheddar Cheese
12 Eggs
6 Oz Heavy Cream
½ tsp Garlic Powder
½ tsp Onion Powder
½ tsp Salt
½ tsp Pepper

Chapter fourteen.
Spaghetti Squash Pancakes

Nutrition Information:

Serves: 2
Serving size: 2 pancakes

Calories: 287

Fat: 18

Carbohydrates: 10

Fiber: 2

Protein: 19

Prep time: 5 mins
Cook time: 15 mins
Total time: 20 mins

Ingredients:

4 Slices Thick Cut Bacon

2 Eggs

284g (10 Oz) Cooked Spaghetti Squash

1 teaspoon Garlic Powder

1 teaspoon Salt

1 teaspoon Pepper

1 teaspoon Onion Powder

30 g (1 Oz) Parmesan Cheese

How To Prepare-

Prepare your spaghetti squash. Get some of them from the food store.

Arrange the stalks and remove any unwanted areas then wash carefully.

 Heat up a pan and begin to Cook the bacon until it   becomes crisp.
It's time to mix the eggs, Spaghetti Squash, spices and cheese in a separate bowl
While stirring to mix other ingredients, add bacon to the mix

Now we need to make four different piles so that we can have our desired recipe. Now scoop some bacon into the pan that already contains bacon grease Cook until the bottom begins to turn brown in colour then flip the other side Serve when it is ready.

Chapter fifteen.
Stuffed Peppers

Nutrition Information:

Serves: 2

Serving size: 1 Pepper

Calories: 484

Fat: 35

Carbohydrates: 14

Fiber: 3

Protein: 30

Prep time: 15 mins
Cook time: 20 mins
Total time: 35 mins

List of Ingredients:

2 Green Peppers

1 Small Onion

2 Sausage Links

1.5 Oz Parmesan Cheese

2 Oz. Cream Cheese

1 Egg

2 Quail Eggs

How To Prepare-

In this recipe, we shall be cutting most vegetables. Now begin to take off the skin of the sausage cook the sausage Remove the seeds from the pepper by cutting it open.

Cut your peppers and onions into small sizes and prepare to cook them. Cook then carefully

Get some parmesan and cut to smaller sizes

Add and mix all the ingredients that have been chopped in a bowl and add cream cheese

Add quail eggs to the peppers and begin to cook for 20 minutes

Chapter sixteen.

Zucchini and Goat Cheese Wraps
Information:

Serves: 6

Serving size: 1 roll

Calories: 186

Fat: 14

Carbohydrates: 3

Fiber: 1

Protein: 13

Prep time: 10 mins
Cook time: 5 mins
Total time: 15 mins

List of Ingredients:

1 Zucchini

6 Oz Soft Goat Cheese

1 tsp dried mint

1 tsp dried dill

Salt and Pepper Oil

How To Prepare-

Remove the ends of the zucchini and wash properly

Now you slice the zucchini into ⅛"
slices

Coat with spices such as oil and pepper

Cook the zucchini on both sides for five minutes

Add and combine with goat milk and cheese

Its easiest to roll the goat cheese into a cylinder between your fingers and then spread it on the zucchini

Roll your already prepared zucchini and put a stick at the centre e.g. toothpick

Chapter seventeen.

Cheesy Sausage Balls

Information:

Serves: 12

Serving size: 1 Ball

Calories: 173

Fat: 14

Carbohydrates: 1
Fiber: 0
Protein: 10.

Prep time: 10 mins
Cook time: 5 mins
Total time: 15 mins

List of Ingredients:

12 oz. Jimmy Dean's Sausage
6 oz. Shredded Cheddar cheese
12 Cubes Cheddar (Optional)

How To Prepare-

Mix shredded cheese and sausage
Divide into 12 equal parts
Place cube of cheese into centre of
sausage and roll into balls
(Optional) Freeze the sausage balls
Fry at 375 degrees until crispy.

Conclusion

This brings us to the end of this
exercise. I sincerely
hope the recipes and method of
application you've
Learned here will help you to achieve the
keto
lifestyle you desire. The opportunities
for weight-loss
and staying healthy are endless, and
you're indeed
poised to participate in this development
if you
implement the use of the
aforementioned recipes
and procedures.
This list of carbohydrate-based foods is
rather lengthy, but that doesn't mean
you will be able to consume all of these
as part of your ketogenic diet. While it is
possible that some people will be able to
reach ketosis eating plenty of the foods

you see on this list, many others must limit their consumption to the green, leafy vegetables on this list or even omit carbs entirely. Again, figure out what your carbohydrate tolerance is first and then choose wisely.

Index

Arugula   Garlic   Radishes
Artichokes   Green beans
        Raspberries
Asparagus   Jicama   Rhubarb
Blackberries   Kale   Scallions
Blueberries   Leeks   Shallots
Bok choy   Lemon   Snow peas

Broccoli   Lettuce   Spaghetti squash
  Brussels sprouts   Lime
        Spinach
  Cabbage   Mushrooms
        Strawberries

Cauliflower   Okra   Summer
squash
 Celery   Onions   Tomatoes
 Chicory greens   Parsley
         Watercress
 Cranberries   Peppers   Wax
beans
 Cucumbers   Pumpkin
      Zucchini
 Eggplant   Radicchio
Proteins
 If you look at the nutritional facts label
and see that a product has 7 grams of
fat and 7 grams of protein, you are good
to go. The higher the percentage of fat
in a food, the better.

Bacon (not turkey bacon)   Kielbasa
 Beef jerky (watch out for added sugars)
       Pepperoni
Beef ribs   Pheasant
Beef roast   Pork chops
Bratwurst   Pork ribs

Chicken (choose the darkest cuts, skin on)   Pork rinds
 Duck   Pork roast
 Eggs (whole)   Quail
 Fish (salmon, bass, carp, flounder, halibut, mackerel, sardines, trout)   Salami
 Ground beef (not lean)   Sausage
 Goose   Shellfish (scallops, shrimp, crab meat, mussels, oysters)
 Ham   Steak (the fatter the better)
 Hot dog (Nathan's brand is the best)   Tuna

Turkey (darker pieces are best)   Veal

Fats

The benefit of ketosis is that it utilises our fat stores and dietary fat as they were meant to be used—for energy.
And finally we come to what is arguably the best part of being on a ketogenic diet—the abundance of delicious,

satisfying, and nutritious fats you can eat!

Almonds   Coconut oil

Almond butter   Cream cheese

Almond milk, unsweetened   Dark chocolate (80 percent or higher)

Almond oil   Fish oil (Carlson brand is a fabulous cod liver oil).

Avocado   Flax seeds and oil (men should probably not consume this because of possible prostate cancer risks)

Avocado oil   Ghee

Beef tallow   Greek yogurt

Blue cheese   Heavy whipping cream

Brazil nuts   Lard

Butter (Kerry gold is a high-quality brand)   Macadamia nut oil

Cheese (cheddar, Colby, feta, mozzarella, provolone, ricotta, Swiss, and others),

Chicken fat, Olive oil,
Coconut   Pecans,
Coconut Cream , Pili nuts,

Coconut milk, unsweetened
Pistachios,
Sour cream,   Sunflower seeds
Walnuts. Your ketogenic diet Keeps
carbs low.
Eat more fat,
Test ketones often.